SKIN CARE BOX

Natural skin care guide and tips

Simple homemade recipes, beauty tips and more

EGERE DEBORAH

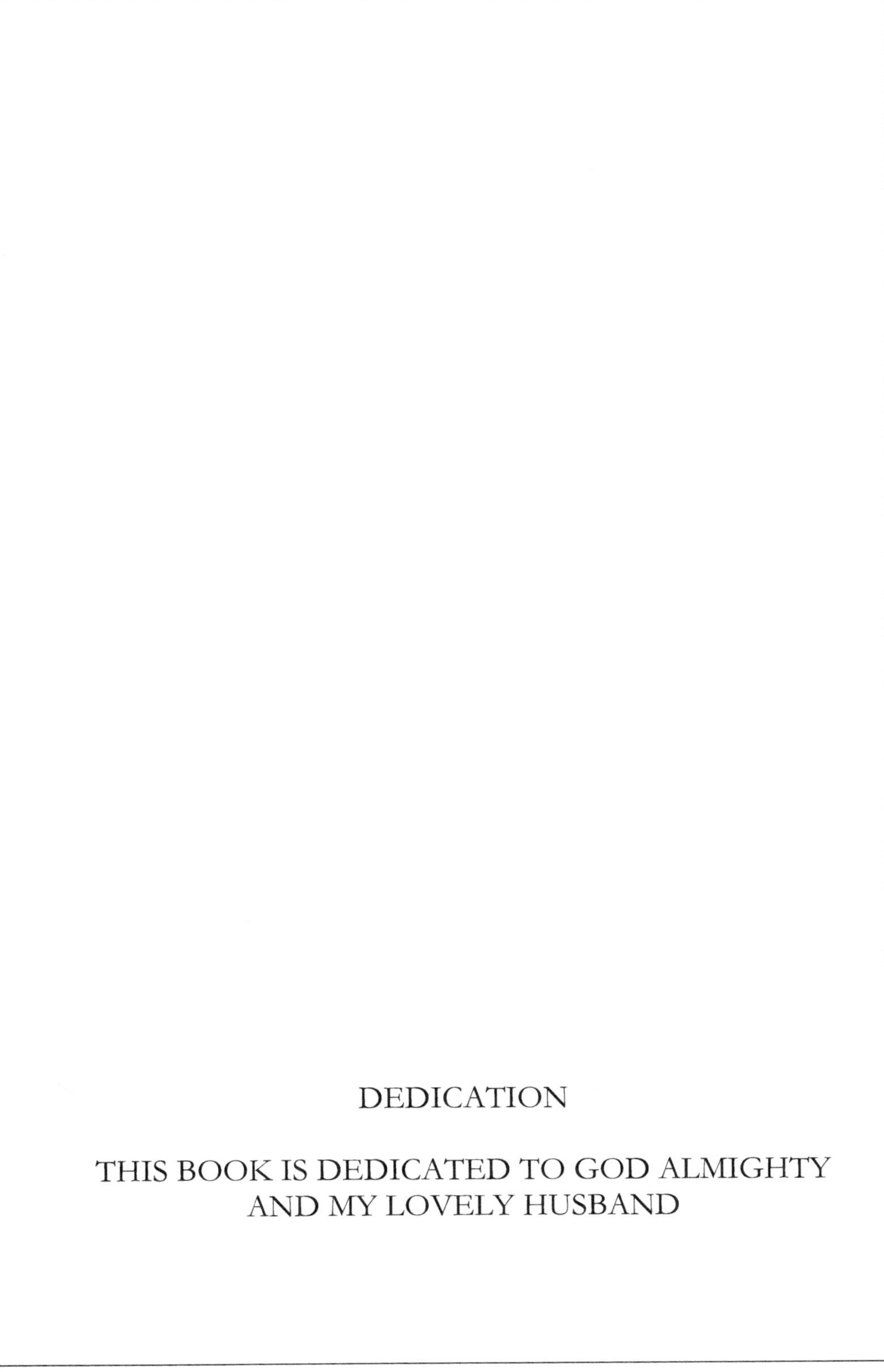

DEDICATION

THIS BOOK IS DEDICATED TO GOD ALMIGHTY
AND MY LOVELY HUSBAND

CONTENTS

INTRODUCTION

Throughout how to make Organic Skincare Recipes, you'll find amazing skincare Products that will take your skin and your mind, body, and spirit to places they've never been before. Filled with all-natural ingredients like fresh herbs Flowers, honey, Shea butter, or a unique essential oil blend, each Recipe allows you to mix up your personalized batch of Skincare that is free of the hazardous chemicals found in store-bought brands. The ingredient has been chosen for the health and beauty benefits of the Ingredients. Each recipe contains step-by-step instructions that teach you how to use oils, herbs, and other organic ingredients to create nourishing products for healthy skin. You will find facial Care treatment plans to help you create a natural beauty routine that's perfect for your unique skin type. These recipes are inspired by the simple things in life that make you feel Alive. From the gorgeous flowers blooming in the garden to the fresh and tangy scent of fresh fruit with A softly scented breeze. Nature provides an amazing world full of therapeutic ingredients for you to create these Exquisite skincare products. Each recipe is organic, natural, and chemical free. Because why would you put something on your body that you shouldn't put in it?

Each one of these replenishing products is special and unique, and they are very easy to create which means they make impressive gifts for holidays, birthdays, or any other special occasion. You can make these skincare Recipes in your kitchen with the tools and ingredients you have on hand. Most of the ingredients can be found at the natural food store or market there are a few specialty ingredients or types of packaging that are easily found online with a quick

Internet search. I formulate these gorgeous recipes with love. It's simply what I do. I hope that Shows. And I hope you will love discovering these creations as much as I enjoyed putting them together for you. I humbly suggest that you make these recipes with focused healing intention and lots of love. Those Two little things are my secret and favorite ingredients and I include them in all of my recipes.

CHAPTER 1

WHAT YOU NEED TO KNOW ABOUT SKIN CARE

Have you ever not washed your face before bed and awakened to a bunch of little pimples? Have you ever eaten a bunch of French fries, chocolate, or junk food and had your skin erupt in an epic breakout the next day or two? Who hasn't? The relationship between your skin and your body is symbiotic, mutually reliant, and interdependent. It is important to realize that the foundation for healthy, radiant skin starts on the inside. Your skin is the largest and fastest-growing organ of your body and accounts for 6 to 10 per cent of your body weight. All of your cells require good nutrition, Proper hydration, oxygenation, and detoxification to thrive. What you put on your skin is just as important as what you put in your body. With this in mind, Healthy skin can be achieved by making positive, well-considered choices concerning your mind, body, and spirit. In addition to your skincare regimen, you want to pay attention to additional factors that can contribute to healthy skin including:

- Sun exposure
- Eating habits
- Hydration
- Exercise
- Environmental pollutants and more …

All of these factors combine with your genetic makeup and

overall wellness to comprise the health of your skin. And while skincare products can help combat and correct some of the inherent issues and skin conditions, it is best to think of Healthy skin holistically, as part of a completely healthy you. After all, a healthy you is a happy you. Keeping that in mind let's take a look at the simple things that make the recipes in this book decadent, healthy, and inspiring!

Throughout this book, you will find recipes that call for fresh fruits, Vegetables, herbs, and flowers. Just like the food you eat these natural skincare Ingredients are best used when fresh. Fresh ingredients are at their peak of Vitality, and plants that are picked at their peak and used immediately will contribute their nutrient-rich vitality to the recipe. You'll also find super foods in quite a few of the skincare recipes due to their high concentrations of vital nutrients that greatly benefit your skin. But no matter which recipe you make, remember that fresh is best!

Make the right size you'll find both single-use and large-batch recipes throughout the book. Most of the single-use recipes are made with fresh, perishable skin food ingredients and are intended to be used immediately. The larger batch recipes can be made ahead of time and used in your daily skincare routine. You'll also find various recipes that make multiples, such as Body Butter that you can creatively package as party favors and gorgeous handmade gifts for your loved ones.

For me, organic is a lifestyle. My skincare company, Debbie's organic skin glow, was founded on organic principles. My main goal when I started my skincare company was to offer consumers highly effective, botanically-based products with incredible natural scents.

The recipes you'll find throughout this book allow you to create your own natural and deliciously scented products in your own home. So, when shopping for the ingredients, keep the quality of the final product in mind. Your creation will only be "organic" if the raw materials you source are organic. Unfortunately, if the ingredient isn't organic, then you can almost certain that it was grown with synthetic fertilizers and pesticides or is a modified ingredient. I make choices to limit my exposure to man-made chemicals in our environment, and I encourage you to do the same. I am a firm believer in the benefits of organic farming for our food and water supply, our skincare products, and the overall health and well-being of our planet Earth and all of its inhabitants.

Many of the skincare recipes in the book will benefit all skin types, and others are intended for specific skin types and conditions. You may wonder how the same facial cleanser could benefit dry, maturing skin and also be good for oily, acne-prone skin. Well, many botanical ingredients are balancers. This means that, as the plant substance makes its way through the bloodstream, it attends to the specific needs of the person. For example, a product can be either calming or stimulating depending on the person who uses it. While this concept is not widely accepted in Western medical philosophy, it has been effectively employed for thousands of years in traditional Chinese medicine, additionally, all skin types benefit from increased cellular health and regeneration. Many of the skincare preparations included in this book are formulated as tonic skin conditioners to promote vitality and support balanced oil production in all skin types.

INTRODUCTION TO SKIN TYPES

Everyone's skin is normal to them, but to care for diverse skin types, we often group people into some skin categories. Ascertaining your skin type is an important first step in knowing how to treat your skin, what products to use, and how to have perfect skin.

- **Step 1**

Wash your face to remove the makeup. Wash with a gentle cleanser and pat dry. This cleans away oils and dirt that may have accumulated during your day, giving your skin a fresh start. Do not over wash though.

- **Step 2**

Wait for 30mins. During this time, your skin should return to its natural state, the characteristics of which will determine your skin type. Act normally and don't touch your face.

- **Step 3**

Dab your face with a tissue. Pay attention to the 'T-zone'- the area of your forehead and nose.

Exfoliation helps to remove dead skin cells, thus boosting tightness. Once or twice a week depending on the skin e.g. Some skins are very close stubborn and have a lot of dead cells which stop creams/soaps to be effective; such skin can exfoliate twice a week.

How to exfoliate: Wet the body with water then use your exfoliating scrub in a circular motion, concentrating more on dark parts or where you have patches on the skin.

Note: For acne/ blemishes face, you can steam (put hot water in a bucket, add disinfectant e.g. Dettol and salt, then hold the water 10 inches away from your face, covering your head with a towel)for like 5 minutes to 10mins.

SKIN TYPES

- Normal
- Oily
- Dry
- Combination.

• NORMAL SKIN

Normal skin shows neither oil nor flaking skin. It should feel supple and smooth. If you have it, consider yourself lucky

• OILY SKIN

Oily skin is characterized by the grease on the tissue. It is also common for a person with oily skin to have large pores and a shine.

• DRY SKIN

Dry skin may feel taut or show flakes of dead skin. It is associated with small pores. Moisturizing is important for this skin type.

- ## COMBINATION SKIN

Skin is the most common. It exhibits traits of all three of the above skin types. Usually, the skin is oily in the T-zone and normal to dry elsewhere.

SIMPLE DAILY ROUTINE YOU MIGHT WANT TO CONSIDER

Your skin will produce more sebum (oil) if it's dehydrated to keep itself lubricated. This can be affected by your environment, the products you use, your stress levels, diet, lifestyle choices and more. One of the most important things you can do for your skin is to stay healthy is to drink more water; your skin is part of you.

HOW TO CONVERT (ML) MEASUREMENT TO (GRAM) MEASUREMENT

Any recipe you see ml… you will know how to measure while using your scale also… Here is another simple method of converting your measurements to the ones suitable for you.

ML TO GRAM

1ml 1gram
2ml 2gram
7ml 7gram
9ml 9gram
50ml 50gram
250ml 250gram

TABLESPOON TO GRAM

1tbs 15gram
2tbs 30gram
5tbs 75gram
7tbs 105gram
8tbs 120gram
10tbs 150gram

GRAMS TO TABLESPOON

10gram 0.78tbs
20gram 1.56tbs
40gram 3.12tbs
90gram 6.34tbs
100gram 7.82tbs
125gram 8.45tbs

TABLESPOON TO ML

1tbs 14.7ml
2tbs 29.57ml
3tbs 44.36ml
5tbs 73.72ml
7tbs 103.51ml
19tbs 280.9ml
20tbs 295.74ml

TABLESPOON TO CUPS

16tbs 1cup
12tbs ¾ cup
10tbs+2tps 2/3 cup
8tbs ½ cup
6tbs 3/8 cup

2tbs 1/8 cup
2tbs+2tps 1/6 cup
3tps 1tbs
4tbs ¼ cup

OUNCE (OZ) TO TABLESPOON

1oz 2tbs
2oz 4tbs
3oz 6tbs
8oz 16tbs
10oz 20tbs
16oz 32tbs

HOW TO CALCULATE PERCENTAGES TO GRAM

6.5/100 * 500=32.5
6.5%is the measurement of that particular product you need in the formulation
100 is what you'll divide all your % with
500 is the size you want to produce
If you want to produce a 1000 size:
6.5/100= 0.065
0.065 * 1000= 65
That's how to calculate in percentage

CHAPTER 2

FACIAL CARE

Taking good care of your facial skin is quite simple when you break it Down to the basics—cleanse, tone, and moisturize your face twice per day, every day. The first step is a cleanser such as gently cleaning the dirt, sweat, oil, and environmental buildup from the surface of your skin to prevent redness, irritation, clogged pores, and dull, ashy skin. Next, you'll use a facial toner to correct the pH level on the surface of your skin and close and minimize your pores so they don't fill up with gunk. The final crucial step is to use a facial moisturizer that will leave your Skin with a nourishing moisture layer that addresses the needs of your specific skin type. Why use a moisturizer? Well, without one, your skin will go haywire trying to overcorrect, causing overly dry or overly oily skin which brings redness, breakouts and clogged pores. Throughout this chapter, you'll find everything you need to follow these three basic steps.

- **VITAMIN C SERUM**

Vitamin C is a powerful antioxidant that can help to improve the appearance of your skin. When you apply vitamin C serum to the affected area, it works by promoting the synthesis of collagen. This is the protein that builds your skin structure and promotes healthy skin. With increased collagen production, the healing of acne wounds is faster.

INGREDIENTS

1 tsp of Vitamin C powder
8 tsp of pure organic rose water
1 tsp of vegetable glycerin
¼ tsp of vitamin E oil
2 drops of lemon essential oil (optional)

DIRECTIONS

1. Dissolve the vitamin C powder in the organic rose water by stirring it with a non-metal spoon until it is fully liquefied. If you have vitamin C Granules.
2. Once fully dissolved, add in the vegetable glycerin and vitamin E oil and stir those in until fully combined.
3. Using a small funnel, transfer your mixture into a dark-tinted glass dropper bottle.
4. Now drop in your essential oil (if using), screw on the lid and shake vigorously to ensure the oil gets mixed.
5. Store in amber bottles

- **ROSE FACE CREAM.**

Rose face creams are eminent for their delicate saturating properties. They sanitize and tone the skin for a brilliant appearance. Additionally, the disinfectant and astringent fixing they contain are likewise calming ingredients.

OIL PHASE.

- 6g of emulsifying wax
- 3g of cetyl alcohol
- 10g macadamia oil
- 5g avocado oil
- 59 rosehip oil

WATER PHASE

- 66g of water
- 2.5g glycerin.

COOLING PHASE.

- 0.5g vitamin E oil
- 0.5g (10drops) lavender essential oil
- 0.5g (10drops) Frankincense oil.
- 1g (drops) Preservative Optiphen.

DIRECTION.

Place the oil phase ingredients in a double boiler and allow ingredients to melt bringing the temperature to 65 -75oc. Boil the kettle water and pour the appropriate amount of water over the glycerin this is from your water phase. Check that both the oil phase and water phase are at the same temperature around 65-75o c. Slowly add the water phase to the oil phase, whisk gently all the time be careful not to introduce too many air bubbles keep stirring for a couple of minutes. Place the bowl containing the cream over the second bowl of cold water and continue to stir as it cools it will start to thicken. Add the preservative and other cooling phase ingredients and mix well. Pour into your container. This should keep for 12 months with preservatives and without preservatives for 1 week, store in the fridge.

- ## **HYALURONIC SERUM**

It helps to keep the skin hydrated and looking young. A serum with hyaluronic acid can improve the appearance of wrinkles and fine lines. It can also help to improve skin tone and texture. Helps to retain moisture in the skin it can also be effective in treating dry skin conditions

INGREDIENTS
- 1tsp of Hyaluronic powder
- ½ cup of Rosewater
- ½ cup of Distilled water
- ½tsp of preservative

- ## **DAY FACE CREAM**

The day face cream is our daily moisturizer; it is so much more than just moisturizing. One of the benefits of the day cream is that it can help reduce or prevent those dreaded wrinkles. If you worry about ageing or the appearance of wrinkles, using a day cream can help to combat it

INGREDIENTS

- 1tsp of Shea butter/cocoa butter/mango butter or coconut oil
- 5-6drops of Rosehips seed oil
- 1tsp of Vitamin E oil
- ½ tsp of Sunscreen

DIRECTION

Melt Shea butter on a double boiler for -60 seconds allow it to cool down for about 5-10minutes then add rosehip oil, vitamin E oil and sunscreen. Allow it to cool down for 5mins to harden then scoop it into a neat Container.

- ## NATURAL SUNSCREEN

They help to prevent sunburn and premature ageing (such as wrinkles, and leathery skin). Sunscreens also help to decrease the risk of skin cancer and also of sunburn-like skin reactions (sun sensitivity) caused by some medications.

INGREDIENTS

- 1tsp Aloe Vera oil
- 1tsp Zinc oxide
- 2tsp coconut oil
- 2tsp Shea butter
- 5 drops of lavender essential oil

DIRECTION

Add everything in a bowl except lavender essential oil, melt on top Of a double boiler, bring it down after melting and allow it to cool. Add 5 drops of lavender essential oil and mix.

- ## **NIGHT FACE CREAM**

A night cream boosts your collagen production, helping your skin to look plumper and firmer. This reduces the appearance of fine lines and wrinkles and lessens sagging. In short, the elasticity of your skin is given a much-needed boost.

INGREDIENTS

- Evening primrose oil – ½ tsp
- Vitamin E oil – ½ tsp
- Avocado oil – 1 tsp
- Shea butter -1tbp

DIRECTION

Melt Shea butter in a double boiler on low heat. Allow cooling after Melting then add primrose oil, avocado oil and vitamin E oil. Mix until it has a lotion look. Note: Always keep your cream away from heat. Allow the cream to soak into your skin for a few minutes before applying makeup. The face cream is a facial moisturizer.

- ## **FACIAL MUD MASK**

Similar to clay masks, mud masks are known for their antibacterial and exfoliating benefits. Mud masks remove impurities from the skin, unclogging pores and absorbing excess oil.

INGREDIENTS

- 1.5 tbsp cooled green tea
- 1 tbsp aloe Vera gel

- 2 tbsp bentonite clay
- ½ tsp argan oil
- 3 drops of geranium essential oil
- Mixing bowl & spoon

DIRECTIONS

1. In a mixing bowl, add 2 tbsp of bentonite clay or any other cosmetic Clay of your choice.
2. Now add 1 tbsp of cooling aloe vera gel and ½ tsp of argan oil and mix well to form a paste.
3. Next, slowly keep adding cooled green tea while stirring well to form an easily spreadable mixture.
4. Finally, add 3 drops of geranium essential oil and stir again. To use apply a facial mud mask onto your clean face and neck. Let it sit For 15 minutes then splash your skin with warm water and remove the mask
Gently with an old washcloth

- **ACTIVATED CHARCOAL PEEL-OFF MASK**

It draws grime, bacteria, oil and other impurities from the skin, which makes it an amazing ingredient to treat all your skin woes.

It's even better when you use an activated charcoal peel-off mask as it exfoliates your skin and sloughs away dead skin cells.

Note: Do not use a metal container or spoon for this face mask. Metal makes the Bentonite clay lose its potency.

INGREDIENTS

- 2 tbsp activated charcoal
- ½ tsp bentonite clay
- 1 tbsp unflavored gelatin powder
- 2 tbsp rose water

- 2 drops of tea tree essential oil
- Shot glass/heat-safe container & non-metal spoon
- Bowl of hot water

DIRECTIONS

1. Empty 2 tbsp of activated charcoal into the shot glass then add the Bentonite clay and unflavored gelatin powder.
2. Pour in the rose water or just plain water, if you want.
3. Now stir well until combined then place the shot glass in the bowl of Hot water to warm and thicken up.
4. Stir it and when it's thick, remove it from the hot water and add the tea Tree essential oil & mix again.
5. Use your clean fingers to apply the mask in a thick even coat, avoiding the area around the eyes do not applying the mask on places where there's hair that you don't want to remove (eyebrows).
6. After the mask dries up completely, the fun part has arrived: time to Peel-off!
 Peel off the mask from one edge coming inwards.
7. After the entire mask is off, wash your face with hot water and a mild cleaner then splash it with cold water.

- **FACE GLOW SERUM**

It absorbs quickly into your skin, Soothes sensitive skin improves the appearance of fine lines and wrinkles, protects your skin from free radicals and future damage, and has the potential to provide more visible results. It feels light on your skin.

INGREDIENTS

- 2 tbsp argan oil

- 2 tbsp rosehip oil
- 2tbsp sesame oil
- 10 drops of lemon essential oil
- 7 drops of geranium essential oil
- Small funnel

DIRECTIONS

1. 4 oz / 1ml amber glass dropper bottle, a small funnel, add 2 tbsp of argan oil, 2 tbsp of rosehip oil and 2 tbsp of sesame oil into your amber glass dropper bottle.
2. Next carefully add 10 drops of lemon essential oil and 7 drops of geranium essential oil.
3. Close the bottle and shake well to mix up all the oils.
4. It can last for more than a year if handled and stored properly without contamination.
5. Use only at night time by massaging about 4 drops all over your clean face.

CHAPTER 3

BODY SCRUBS

A large part of the human experience is the act of bathing, becoming clean again. We shower to invigorate, wake up and face the day. We Wash off the day's work or play. We wash to primp and preen ourselves for social events. And we have learned to create little slices of sensory Heaven within this daily experience by bringing scent, texture, and luxury to the bath and shower by using body washes and body scrubs that Combine soap, exfoliation, and moisturizer into one amazing product. A wide variety of nutritious exfoliating ingredients are Combined with botanical oils and essential oils for benefits to the mind, body, and spirit. After all, who wants to wash with just soap when you can use a body scrub this chapter is guaranteed to turn an ordinary shower into an extraordinary home spa experience!

- **COCONUT SCRUB**

Using a coconut body scrub is both relaxing, good for your skin and helps maintain the natural chemical balance of the skin while softening and helping to alleviate dryness.

INGREDIENTS

- Coconut oil-76g
- Sheabutter-32g
- Ewax-8.75g
- Cetyl alcohol-6.25g
- Rose petals-0.88g

- Rosehip seed oil-0.63g
- Strawberry extract-0.63g
- Germall plus preservative -0.63g
- Sugar- 200g

DIRECTIONS

Double boil the base (coconut oil, Shea butter, e-wax, cetyl) on low heat, and put it in the refrigerator to freeze (50% solid and 50% liquid), bring it out after it has solidified a little, whip for some time, and add in your cool-down phase (Rosehip seed oil, strawberry extract, gaermallplus, whip a little then add your sugar whip till it becomes fluffy then transfer into your containers.

- ## COFFEE SCRUB

Coffee scrub is great at cleaning the skin Soothes Your Skin, Offers Skin Tightening Properties, Improves Circulation, Fights Aging, Reduces Cellulite and Makes Your Skin Glow.

INGREDIENTS

- Sheabutter- 32g
- Avocado oil- 33g
- Sunflower oil- 33g
- E-wax- 8.75g
- Cetyl alcohol- 6.25g
- Sugar-200g
- Coffee-100h
- Germallplus-0.639

DIRECTIONS

Double boil the base (Avocado oil, Shea butter, e-wax, cetyl alcohol, sunflower oil) on low heat, put it in the refrigerator to freeze (50% solid and 50% liquid), and bring it out after it has solidified a little, whip for some time, after whipping add in germallplus whip a little then add your sugar and coffee, whip till it becomes fluffy then transfer into your containers.

- ## TURMERIC SCRUB

Turmeric is an antibacterial agent. Turmeric scrub helps to heal acne and lightens skin and helps delay ageing. It is extremely moisturizing for the body. It makes skin smooth, soft and glowing and suits most skin types.

INGREDIENTS

- Base
- Turmeric butter- 32g
- Shea butter- 32g
- Sunflower oil- 30g
- E-wax- 8.75g
- Cool down phase
- Turmeric essential oil-2 tablespoon
- Lemon essential oil-1 tablespoon
- Bergamot essential oil-1 tablespoon
- Turmeric powder- 2 tablespoon
- Vitamin E-1teaspoon
- Liquid germallplus-0.63g
- Sugar-200g

DIRECTIONS

Double boil the base (sunflower oil, Shea butter, e-wax,

turmeric butter) on low heat, put it in the refrigerator to freeze (50% solid and 50% liquid), bring it out after it has solidified a little, and whip for some time add in your cool-down phase (turmeric Essential oil, lemon essential oil, bergamot essential oil, turmeric powder, vitamin E, gaermallplus), whip a little then add your sugar whip till it becomes fluffy then transfer into your containers.

• MINT SUGAR SCRUB

Mint can be used on any skin type and is especially good for oily and combination skin because it helps balance natural oils. That means fewer clogged pores. Peppermint essential oil has a cool, minty scent that promotes blood flow and helps liven the feeling of your skin.

INGREDIENTS

- Sunflower oil- ¼ cup
- Safflower oil- ¼
- Avocado oil-¼
- Cranberry seeds-2tablespoon
- Peppermint essential oil-1tablespoon
- Lemon grass essential oil-1tablespoon
- Beewax- 6.25g
- Emulsifying wax-8.75g
- Sugar- 4cup
- Germallplus-½teaspoon

DIRECTION

Double boil the base (Avocado oil, beeswax, e-wax, sunflower oil, sunflower oil) on low heat put it in the refrigerator to freeze (50% solid and 50% liquid), and bring it out after it has solidified a little whip for some time after whipping add in your essential oils, germallplus whip a little then add your sugar and cranberry seeds and whip till it becomes fluffy then transfer them into your containers.

• TEA TREE SCRUB

This body scrub is an excellent choice for people who have a spot or acne-prone skin. Tea Tree is well known for its excellent antimicrobial, antiseptic and antifungal properties. Use this and your skin will feel smooth, soft and deeply moisturized.

INGREDIENTS

- Avocado oil - ¼
- Sunflower oil- ¼
- Tee tree essential oil- 2tablespoon
- Lemon grass essential oil- 2table spoon
- Beewax- 6.25g
- Emulsifying wax-8.75g
- Neem powder-2table spoon
- Sugar-4cup
- Germallplus-½

DIRECTION

Double boil the base (Avocado oil, beeswax, e-wax, sunflower oil) on low heat put it in the refrigerator to freeze (50% solid and 50% liquid), and bring it out after it has solidified a little whip for some time after whipping add in your essential oils, germallplus whip a little then add your sugar and Neem powder whip till it becomes fluffy then transfer it into your containers.

- ## **GRAPEFRUIT SUGAR SCRUB**

It contains a high amount of Vitamins A and C and is loaded with minerals and antioxidants that can help protect your skin from environmental hazards and even stimulates the production of collagen, leaving your skin toned and smooth.

INGREDIENTS

- Sunflower oil-¼cup
- Safflower oil -¼cup
- Avocado oil-¼cup
- Rose clay-1tablespoon
- Sugar-4cup
- Grapefruit essential oil- 2tablespoon
- Bee wax-6.25g
- Emulsifying wax-8.75g

DIRECTION

Double boil the base (Avocado oil, beeswax, e-wax, sunflower) on low heat put it in the refrigerator to freeze (50% solid and 50% liquid), and bring it out after it has solidified a little whip for some time after whipping add in your essential oils, germallplus whip a little then add your sugar and rose clay whip till it becomes fluffy then transfer into your containers.

CHAPTER 4

SOAP MAKING

Soap is a substance used with water for washing and cleaning dirt and also helps exfoliate the skin; it is made up of a compound of natural oils or fats with sodium hydroxide or another strong alkali.

• TURMERIC AND LEMON SOAP

This soap is a perfect combo for acne and brightens up those dark spots, which leave you with smooth, even-toned skin that glows.

INGREDIENTS

- Shea butter-200g
- Coconut oil-200g
- Olive oil-300g
- Castor oil-200g
- Palm oil-200g
- Sodium hydroxide-300g
- Water and Ice-300g (50% water -50% ice)
- Turmeric powder-15g
- Lemon peel-15g
- Liquorice powder-15g
- Lemon essential oil-15g

DIRECTION

Before you start making your product always put on your safety goggles and neoprene gloves

1. Place your sodium hydroxide also known as lye in a container add your water and ice while stirring gradually, and stir well till dissolved. Set aside to cool down (80 degrees Fahrenheit to 100 degrees Fahrenheit).
2. Combine your butter and oil and heat gently, when dissolved set aside to cool down a bit.

3. Mix your powders and your essential oil.

4. Pour your lye solution into your melted oil and stick the blend after that add your powders and essential oil solution to it stick the blend very well after mixing everything pour it into your moulder and allow it to solidify night after that you can cut your soap into sizes.

• OAT AND HONEY SOAP

This is perfect for all skin types. It is gentle and it will help clear all blemishes and soothe irritated dry skin leaving the skin smooth and moisturized

INGREDIENTS

- Shea butter-200g
- Coconut oil-200g
- Olive oil-300g
- Castor oil-200g
- Palm oil-200
- Sodium hydroxide-300g
- Water and ice-300g (50%water-50%ice)
- Colloidal oat-50g
- Raw honey-50g

DIRECTION

Before you start making your product always put on your safety goggles and neoprene gloves

1. Place your sodium hydroxide also known as lye in a container and add your water and ice while stirring gradually stir well till dissolved. Set aside to cool down (80 degrees Fahrenheit to 100 degrees Fahrenheit).

2. Combine your butter and oil and heat gently when dissolve set aside to cool down a bit.

3. Mix your powders and your essential oil.

4. Pour your lye solution into your melted oil and stick blend after that add your oat powder and Raw honey in it stick the blend very well after mixing everything pour it into your moulder and allow it to solidify overnight after that you can cut your soap into sizes.

• ALOE VERA AND CUCUMBER SOAP

Aloe vera & cucumber is the perfect duo for hydrating and soothing skin, especially for those with sensitive skin. This soap helps with the breakout while keeping your skin smooth and moisturized.

INGREDIENTS

- Sheabutter-1.5 ounce
- Coconut oil- 7.5 ounce
- Olive oil- 7.5ounce
- Castor oil- 1.5ounce
- Palm oil- 7ounce
- Sodium hydroxide- 3.6ounce
- Water and ice- 6.4 ounce (50%-water &50% -ice)
- Fresh cucumber- 5ounce
- Fresh Aloe Vera- 5ounce
- Eucalyptus essential oil-1tablespoon

DIRECTION

Before you start making your product always put on your safety goggles and neoprene gloves

1. Place your sodium hydroxide also known as lye in a container and add your water and ice while stirring gradually stir well till dissolved. Set aside to cool down (80 degrees Fahrenheit to 100 degrees Fahrenheit).

2. Combine your butter and oil and heat gently when dissolve set aside to cool down a bit.

3. Blend your cucumber and aloe Vera.

4. Pour your lye solution into your melted oil and stick blend after that add your cucumber and Aloe Vera in it stick blend very well add the essential oil in and stick blend a little after mixing everything pour it into your moulder and allow it to solidify overnight after that you can cut your soap into sizes.

- **CARROT SOAP**

This soap is perfect for sensitive skin it gently cleanses and exfoliates it, helps get rid of skin infections such as acne, dark spot & many other skin irritation.

INGREDIENTS

- Shea butter- 2.5ounce
- Coconut oil-6.5ounce
- Olive oil-6.5
- Castor oil-1ounce
- Palm oil-5.2 ounce
- Fresh carrot-7ounce
- Poppyseed-1tablespoon
- Sodium hydroxide-3ounce
- Water and ice-6ounce (50% water & 50% ice)

DIRECTION

Before you start making your product always put on your safety goggles and neoprene gloves

1. Place your sodium hydroxide also known as lye in a container add your water and ice while stirring gradually, and stir well till dissolved. Set aside to cool down (80

degrees Fahrenheit to 100 degrees Fahrenheit).

2. Combine your butter and oil and heat gently when dissolve set aside to cool down a bit.

3. Blend your carrot

4. Pour your lye solution into your melted oil and stick blend after that add your carrot juice in it stick blend very well add in your poppy seed and stick blend a little after mixing everything pour it into your moulder and allow it to solidify overnight after that you can cut your soap into sizes.

- **GRAPE FRUIT SOAP**

This soap will give you deep cleansing and also glow your skin leaving your skin well moisturized.

INGREDIENTS

- Sheabutter-1.8ounce
- Coconut oil-9ounce
- Olive oil-14ounce
- Castor oil-1.7ounce
- Palm oil-9ounce
- Grapefruit oil-1.7ounce
- Rose clay-2tablespoon
- Water and ice-10ounce (50%water50%ice)
- Sodium hydroxide-5ounce

DIRECTION

Before you start making your product always put on your safety goggles and neoprene gloves

1. Place your sodium hydroxide also known as lye in a

container and add your water and ice while stirring gradually stir well till dissolved. Set aside to cool down (80 degrees Fahrenheit to 100 degrees Fahrenheit).

2. Combine your butter and oil and heat gently when dissolve set aside to cool down a bit.

3. Measure your rose clay and put it aside.

4. Pour your lye solution into your melted oil and stick blend very well add in your rose clay and stick blend a little after mixing everything pours into your moulder and allow it to solidify overnight after that you can cut your soap into sizes.

- **NEEM &TEA TREE SOAP**

This soap clears acne, scar pigmentation, and blackheads, leaving your skin glowing and smooth.

INGREDIENTS

- Sheabutter-1.8ounce
- Coconut oil-9ounce
- Olive oil-14ounce
- Palm oil-9ounce
- Sodium hydroxide-5.1ounce
- Water and ice-10.2ounce
- Neem powder-2table spoon
- Tea tree essential oil-2 ounce

DIRECTION

Before you start making your product always put on your safety goggles and neoprene gloves.

1. Place your sodium hydroxide also known as lye in a container and add your water and ice while stirring gradually stir well till dissolved. Set aside to cool down (80

degrees Fahrenheit to 100 degrees Fahrenheit).

2. Combine your butter and oil and heat gently when dissolve set aside to cool down a bit.

3. Measure your tea tree essential oil and Neem Powder and put them aside.

4. Pour your lye solution into your melted oil and stick blend very well add in your tea tree essential oil, Neem Powder and stick blend a little after mixing everything pour it into your moulder and allow it to solidify after that you can cut your soap into sizes.

- ## **CHAMOMILE & CALENDULA SOAP**

It helps clear blemishes away, lightens blemishes and soothes irritated skin and also gives your skin a glow.

INGREDIENTS

- Sheabutter-1.8 ounce
- Coconut oil-9ounce
- Olive oil-14ounce
- Castor oil-1.7ounce
- Palm oil-9ounce
- Sodium hydroxide-5ounce
- Water &ice-10ounce (50%water50%ice)
- Chamomile flowers-1ounce
- Calendula flowers-1ounce

DIRECTION

Before you start making your product always put on your safety goggles and neoprene gloves.

1. Place your sodium hydroxide also known as lye in a container and add your water and ice while stirring gradually stir well till dissolved. Set aside to cool down (80

degrees Fahrenheit to 100 degrees Fahrenheit).

2. Combine your butter and oil and heat gently when dissolve set aside to cool down a bit.

3. Measure your chamomile flowers and calendula flowers and put them aside.

4. Pour your lye solution into your melted oil and stick blend very well add in your chamomile flowers, calendula flowers and stick blend a little after mixing everything pour it into your moulder and allow it to solidify overnight after that you can cut your soap into sizes.

- **CHARCOAL & MINT SOAP**

This soap will detoxify the toxins from your skin and it also controls oily skin, giving a cool and relaxed feeling.

INGREDIENTS

- Shea butter-1.8ounce
- Coconut oil-9ounce
- Olive oil-14ounce
- Castor oil-1.7ounce
- Palm oil-9ounce
- Sodium hydroxide-5.1ounce
- Activated charcoal-1ounce
- Peppermint oil-1ounce
- Rosemary essential oil-1ounce
- Water and ice-10ounce (50%water50%ice)

DIRECTION

Before you start making your product always put on your safety goggles and neoprene gloves.

1. Place your sodium hydroxide also known as lye in a container, add your water and ice while stirring gradually,

and stir well till dissolved. Set aside to cool down (80 degrees Fahrenheit to 100 degrees Fahrenheit).
2. Combine your butter and oil and heat gently, when dissolved set aside to cool down a bit.
3. Measure and mix the activated charcoal, peppermint essential oil, and rosemary essential oil, and put them aside.
4. Pour your lye solution into your melted oil and stick blend, stick blend very well add in your mixed essential oils and activated charcoal and stick blend a little, after mixing everything pour it into your moulder and allow it to solidify night after that you can cut your soap into sizes.

- **CITRUS SOAP**

This soap helps in combating problems such as wrinkles, acne, and dark spots leaving your skin glowing and feeling refreshed.

INGREDIENTS

- Sheabutter-2.1ounce
- Coconut oil-7ounce
- Olive oil-7ounce
- Castor oil-1.7ounce
- Palm oil-6ounce
- Sodium hydroxide-4ounce
- Water and ice-8ounce (50%water50%ice)
- Orange essential oil-1ounce
- Grapefruit essential oil-1ounce
- Lemon essential oil-1ounce
- Lime essential oil-1ounce
- Calendula flowers-1ounce

DIRECTION

Before you start making your product always put on your

safety goggles and neoprene gloves.

1. Place your sodium hydroxide also known as lye in a container, add your water and ice while stirring gradually, and stir well till dissolved. Set aside to cool down (80 degrees Fahrenheit to 100 degrees Fahrenheit.

2. Combine your butter and oil and heat gently, when dissolved set aside to cool down a bit.

3. Measure and mix your calendula flower and essential oils and put them aside.

4. Pour your lye solution into your melted oil and stick blend very well add in your mixed essential oils and Calendula flowers stick blend a little after mixing everything pour it into your moulder and allow it to solidify the night after that you can cut your soap into sizes.

- **LAVENDER SOAP**

This soap helps in soothe and calm the skin, combat acne, lightens dark spots and minimizes wrinkles.

INGREDIENTS

- Shea butter-2.1ounce
- Coconut oil-7ounce
- Olive oil-7ounce
- Castor oil-1.7ounce
- Palm oil-6ounce
- Sodium hydroxide-4ounce
- Water and ice-8ounce (50%water50%ice)
- Lavender essential oil-1ounce
- Lavender buds-1ounce

DIRECTION

Before you start making your product always put on your

safety goggles and neoprene gloves.
1. Place your sodium hydroxide also known as lye in a container and add your water and ice while stirring gradually stir well till dissolved. Set aside to cool down (80 degrees Fahrenheit to 100 degrees Fahrenheit
2. Combine your butter and oil and heat gently when dissolve set aside to cool down a bit.
3. Measure your lavender buds and lavender essential oil and put them aside.
4. Pour your lye solution into your melted oil and stick blend very well add in your essential oil and lavender buds stick blend a little after mixing everything pour it into your moulder and allow it to solidify overnight after that you can cut your soap into sizes.

CHAPTER 5

BODY BUTTER

Body butter is a thick cream that is deeply moisturizing. It can help you protect your skin from dryness as well as rough or patchy skin. Body butter typically contains a combination of naturally derived butter like cocoa butter, Shea butter or mango butter.

- ### LAVENDER AND TEA TREE BODY BUTTER

This cream is used for the skin [body &face] that, in addition to moisturizing reduces inflammation, lightens scars, fades dark spots, speeds wound healing and soothes all skin conditions, including rosacea, eczema, psoriasis & dermatitis.

INGREDIENTS

- Shea butter-33.5%
- Mango butter-15%
- Hemp oil-32%
- Jojoba oil-17%
- Vitamin E-1%
- Lavender oil-5%
- Tea tree oil-5%
- Arrowroot powder-5%

DIRECTION

Melt the mango butter and Shea butter over low heat. Mix in the oils and essential oils. Pour the mixture into the bowl of a stand mixer or a bowl that you can use a hand mixer in. Freeze for 30mins when solid, whip for about 10 minutes or until it looks fluffy. When fluffy transfer into your containers.

• COCO BODY BUTTER

Cocoa butter contains a high amount of fatty acids, which makes it the primary ingredient in skin cream. Fatty acids help to hydrate the skin. The fat in cocoa butter protects the skin, holds in moisture and prevents your skin from drying.

INGREDIENTS

- Coco butter-18%
- Shea butter-15%
- Mango butter-15%
- Sunflower oil-15%
- Coconut oil-9%
- Grape seed oil-9%
- Apricot oil-9%
- Olive oil-9%

DIRECTION

Melt the cocoa butter, mango butter and Shea butter over low heat. Mix in the oils. Pour the mixture into the bowl of a stand mixer or a bowl that you can use a hand mixer in a Freezer for 30mins. When solid, whip for about 10 minutes or until it looks fluffy. When fluffy transfer into your containers.

• GLOW BODY BUTTER

The glowing body butter moisturizes and nourishes the

skin. It also protects and treats the skin from skin discoloration psoriasis and eczema, leaving your skin smooth and glowing

INGREDIENTS

- Shea butter-55%
- Jojoba oil-42%
- Almond oil-42%
- Vitamin E oil-2%
- Fragrance oil-2%
- Arrowroot-1%

DIRECTION

Melt the Shea butter over low heat. Mix in the oils. Pour the mixture into the bowl of a stand mixer or a bowl that you can use a hand mixer in a Freezer for 30mins. When solid, whip for about 10 minutes or until it looks fluffy. Add in your vitamin E oil, fragrance and arrowroot powder, and mix until fluffy. When fluffy transfer into your containers.

- ## REFORM BODY BUTTER

This Body Butter is specially formulated for those with Eczema, Psoriasis - sensitive and dry skin. Its infusion of herbs and oils has properties that can help reduce irritation and calm itching. Its main component is Shea butter which has anti-inflammatory and healing properties.

INGREDIENTS

- Chamomile flowers-3tbsp
- Calendula flower-3tbsp
- Marshmallow root-1tbsp

- Shea butter-2cup
- Avocado oil-½cup
- Jojoba oil-½cup
- Hempseed oil-½cup
- Vitamin E oil-3tablespoon

DIRECTION

Melt the Shea butter over low heat. Mix in the herbs-infused oils. Pour the mixture into the bowl of a stand mixer or a bowl that you can use a hand mixer in a Freezer for 30mins. When solid, whip for about 10 minutes or until it looks fluffy. Add in your vitamin E oil, and mix until fluffy. When fluffy transfer into your containers.

- **ECZEMA REFORM BODY BUTTER**

This Body Butter is for those with Eczema, Psoriasis - sensitive and dry skin. Its infusion of herbs and oils has properties that can help reduce irritation and calm itching. Its main component, Shea Butter, is known for its anti-inflammatory and healing properties.

INGREDIENTS

- Chamomile flowers-3tbsp
- Calendula flower-3tbsp
- St John wort -1tbsp
- Shea butter-2cup
- Avocado oil-½cup
- Jojoba oil-½cup
- Vitamin E oil-3tablespoon
- Arrowroot powder-1tbsp

DIRECTION

Melt the Shea butter over low heat. Mix in the herbs-infused oils. Pour the mixture into the bowl of a stand mixer or a bowl that you can use a hand mixer in a Freezer for 30mins. When solid, whip for about 10 minutes or until it looks fluffy. Add in your vitamin E oil and arrowroot powder, and mix until fluffy. When fluffy transfer into your containers.

CHAPTER 6

BODY OIL

Body oil hydrates and moisturizes dehydrated skin. Improve the texture of the skin. Help the appearance of scars and stretch marks. Improve sleep at night.

- **GLOWING BODY OIL**

INGREDIENTS

- Jojoba oil-12%
- Sunflower oil-50%
- Grape seed oil-35%
- Vitamin E oil-1%
- Fragrance-1%

DIRECTION

Mix all oils, vitamin E oil and fragrance together mix very well then pour into your containers.

- **MOISTURIZING BODY OIL**

INGREDIENTS

- Sunflower oil-53.55g
- Avocado oil-40.85g
- Castor oil-6.3g
- Fragrance-4.2g

DIRECTION

Mix all oils, vitamin E oil and fragrance together mix very well then pour into your containers.

CHAPTER 7

INFUSED BODY OIL

The infused oil has all of the beautiful benefits. Health benefits for the skin can be antiseptic, anti-fungal, calming and relaxing properties. This infused oil soothes psoriasis and other inflammatory conditions.

- ## CHAMOMILE AND CALENDULA BODY OIL

Chamomile and calendula possess many powerful skin properties such as anti-inflammatory, anti-fungal, antibacterial and antiseptic. Additionally, this oil is hypoallergenic and helps to reduce skin irritants by neutralizing free radicals.

INGREDIENTS

- Avocado oil
- Sunflower oil
- Vitamin E oil
- Safflower oil
- Calendula flowers
- Chamomile flowers

DIRECTION

- Prepare your jar.

- Fill the jar with herbs.
- Pour oil over the herbs slowly.
- Cover the jar, give it a few shakes, and put it in a cool place it inside your house
- Cork and label your bottles.

- **LEMON GRASS-INFUSED BODY OIL**

Because Lemongrass has soothing properties, it is commonly used for massage. The refreshing aroma combined with the oil soothing properties make it a popular choice for massage therapy. It also holds purifying benefits for the skin; it also helps in tightening the skin.

INGREDIENTS

- Avocado oil
- Sunflower oil
- Vitamin E oil
- Safflower oil
- Rosemary essential oil
- Lemongrass essential oil

DIRECTION

- Prepare your jar.
- Fill the jar with herbs.
- Pour oil over the herbs slowly.
- Cover the jar, give it a few shakes, and put it in a cool

- Place inside your house.
- Cork and label your bottles.

CONCLUSION

It is a great experience to try new things. If you haven't tried to Do It yourself, it is best that you try this interesting hobby now. We hope this Book has been your handy guide in light on the different corners of organic skincare products and guided you on how to start, how to proceed and how to create visually appealing and beautifully organic skincare products that exfoliate or Nourish your skin. Moreover, we have used a handful of recipes so that you can start right away with recipes from a trusted source. Don't be afraid to get Creative with new ingredients, color patterns, designs and decorations. Making organic skincare products is just like cooking. The possibilities are endless. Set your creativity free and explore.

ABOUT THE AUTHOR

Egere Deborah is a seasoned chemist, who found passion in skincare products and has strong talent for blending organic ingredients to create an effective skin treatment that are sensory journey for the body and this has remain her passion for years.